LISA R. ASHLEY

ZERO POINT RECIPES AND FOOD LIST

The Ultimate Cookbook and Secret Guide to Effortlessly Reduce Weight and Boost Energy (14-Day Meal-Plan Included)

Contents

1

Introduction

Before we begin, let me share the success story of my dear friend Ashley. She is a vibrant, talented individual with a heart of gold, but she carried a burden that she hid beneath her infectious laughter and warm smiles – the weight of her own insecurities. The constant struggle with her body image had taken a toll on Ashley, affecting not only her physical health but also casting shadows on the brilliance that radiated from within her.

One day, as we sat in our favourite coffee shop, sipping on our steaming cups of comfort, I shared with Ashley the transformative journey I had undertaken with the Zero Point Lifestyle. Knowing her struggles, I spoke not of diets, restrictions, or rigorous workout routines, but of a way of life that celebrated food, flavour, and most importantly, self-love.

I vividly remember the spark in Ashley's eyes as I narrated my experience – the joy of discovering delicious recipes, the freedom from counting every calorie, and the empowerment that came with understanding that nourishing our bodies is a beautiful act of self-care. The conversation wasn't about numbers on a scale; it was about embracing a lifestyle that allowed us to savour every bite without guilt, to relish flavours without fear, and to build a relationship with food that was rooted in balance.

As I spoke, I could see a subtle shift in Ashley's perspective. The idea of a lifestyle that didn't demand sacrifice but instead encouraged mindful choices resonated with her. She listened intently, absorbing the essence of a journey that wasn't about shedding pounds but about gaining a profound sense of well-being.

Over the weeks that followed, Ashley tentatively dipped her toes into the world of zero point cooking. Together, we explored recipes that were not only delicious but also satisfying – meals that nourished her body and lifted her spirit. The kitchen became a haven, a space where Ashley discovered the therapeutic joy of preparing meals that were both health-conscious and delectable.

As time unfolded, Ashley's insecurities began to wane. The numbers on the scale became secondary to the vibrant energy she felt, the newfound confidence that emanated from her, and the sense of empowerment that came with making choices that honoured her well-being. The Zero Point Lifestyle had become a compass guiding her towards self-acceptance and a deeper appreciation for the incredible person she was.

Ashley's journey is a testament to the transformative power of the Zero Point Lifestyle. It's not just about what we eat; it's about how we nourish our bodies, celebrate our individuality, and cultivate a positive relationship with ourselves. The Zero Point Lifestyle isn't a quick fix – it's a journey of self-discovery, flavour exploration, and the unwavering belief that every bite is a step towards a healthier, happier life.

And so, the story of Ashley unfolds as she continues to embrace the Zero Point Lifestyle – a story of self-love, resilience, and the profound understanding that the most beautiful journey is the one we take towards becoming the best version of ourselves.

Welcome to the world of Zero Point Cooking, where the journey to wellness is guided by the simplicity and nutritional richness of zero-point foods. In this culinary adventure, we invite you to explore a transformative approach to eating that not only enhances flavour but also promotes a healthy lifestyle.

Understanding the Concept of Zero-Point Foods

Zero-point foods are the backbone of various weight management programs, such as Weight Watchers, offering a revolutionary perspective on mindful and balanced eating. These foods are assigned a point value of zero, allowing you to enjoy them without the need for meticulous counting or tracking. Primarily consisting of nutrient-dense options like fruits, vegetables, lean proteins, and more, zero-point foods provide a foundation for building meals that are not only satisfying but also supportive of your overall well-being.

As you embark on this culinary journey, it's essential to comprehend the essence of zero-point foods. Unlike traditional dieting approaches that focus solely on restriction, zero-point cooking encourages a positive and empowering relationship with food. It promotes the enjoyment of a diverse array of ingredients without the fear of exceeding a predetermined point limit. This paradigm shift from limitation to abundance sets the stage for a sustainable and enjoyable approach to nourishing your body.

How Zero-Point Foods Contribute to a Healthy Lifestyle

Beyond the simplicity of counting points, zero-point foods play a vital role in fostering a holistic and healthy lifestyle. They are the building blocks of nutritious meals that fuel your body with essential vitamins, minerals, and antioxidants. Incorporating these foods into your daily diet offers a plethora of benefits, including:

1. Nutrient Density

Zero-point foods are often rich in essential nutrients, providing your body with the fuel it needs to function optimally. From leafy greens packed with vitamins to lean proteins supporting muscle health, these foods contribute to a well-rounded and balanced nutritional profile.

2. Weight Management

The concept of zero points empowers you to make choices based on nutritional value rather than calorie counting. This approach can be instrumental in weight management, allowing you to focus on the quality of your food rather than strictly adhering to numerical constraints.

3. Flexibility and Variety

Embracing zero-point cooking opens up a world of culinary possibilities. With an expansive list of zero-point foods, you have the flexibility to experiment with various flavours, textures, and cuisines. This not only adds excitement to your meals but also prevents monotony in your diet.

4. Mindful Eating

Zero-point cooking encourages a mindful approach to eating. By savouring and appreciating the flavours of wholesome ingredients, you develop a deeper connection with your food. This mindful awareness can lead to healthier eating habits and a greater appreciation for the nourishment your meals provide.

5. Sustainable Lifestyle Changes

Unlike fad diets that often lead to temporary results, zero-point cooking promotes sustainable lifestyle changes. By incorporating these principles into your daily routine, you create a lasting foundation for health and well-being.

In the pages that follow, you'll discover a treasure trove of zero-point recipes designed to tantalise your taste buds while aligning with your health and fitness goals. From vibrant breakfasts to hearty dinners and delectable desserts, each recipe is crafted to showcase the incredible variety and deliciousness that zero-point cooking has to offer.

So, let the culinary exploration begin! Dive into the recipes, savour the flavours, and embrace a lifestyle where nourishing your body is a

joyous and fulfilling experience. Welcome to Zero Point Cooking –
where every bite is a step toward a healthier, happier you.

2

Chapter 1: What are Zero Point Foods?

Exploring the World of Zero Point Foods

Zero Point Foods, the heart and soul of weight management programs like Weight Watchers, are a culinary revelation that empowers individuals to make health-conscious choices without the constraints of traditional calorie counting. But what exactly qualifies as a zero-point food? In essence, these are nutrient-dense, whole foods that are assigned a point value of zero within specific dietary programs. These foods often include a spectrum of fruits, vegetables, lean proteins, and more.

As we delve into the exploration of zero-point foods, it's essential to recognize that this concept transcends mere point values. Zero-point foods are the nutritional powerhouses that form the foundation of a balanced and mindful eating approach. Understanding their composition, benefits, and the culinary possibilities they offer is key to unlocking a world of flavorful and healthful meals.

How Weight Watchers and Similar Programs Classify Zero Point Foods

Weight Watchers, among other similar programs, has meticulously curated lists of zero-point foods based on their nutritional content and overall health impact. These foods are chosen not just for their absence of points but for their positive contribution to a well-rounded diet. The classification process takes into account factors such as calorie density, nutritional density, and their role in promoting satiety and overall health.

Navigating the intricacies of how zero-point foods are classified offers a roadmap for creating meals that align with the principles of these programs. From colourful vegetables to lean proteins, each zero-point food plays a specific role in building meals that are satisfying, nourishing, and supportive of your health and wellness journey.

Why Zero Points? Understanding the Benefits

The Role of Zero Point Foods in Weight Management

The concept of zero points is not merely a numeric value; it's a strategic approach to weight management that encourages a balanced and flexible dietary lifestyle. Zero-point foods act as the cornerstone of this approach by providing a framework for constructing meals that are not only satisfying but also conducive to weight loss or maintenance.

By incorporating these foods into your daily meals, you create a foundation that allows for flexibility in your overall dietary patterns. This flexibility, in turn, fosters a sustainable and enjoyable approach to weight management. Rather than focusing solely on restriction, the emphasis shifts towards making informed and health-conscious choices.

Nutritional Benefits and Health Advantages

Beyond their role in weight management, zero-point foods offer a host of nutritional benefits that contribute to overall health and well-being. These benefits include:

1. Nutrient Density

Zero-point foods are often rich in essential nutrients such as vitamins, minerals, and antioxidants. Choosing a variety of nutrient-dense foods supports your body's optimal functioning and helps meet daily nutritional requirements.

2. Caloric Consciousness

The emphasis on zero points encourages a mindful awareness of caloric intake. By choosing foods with zero points, you naturally gravitate towards options that are lower in calories, promoting a balanced and calorie-conscious approach to eating.

3. Satiety and Satisfaction

Many zero-point foods are known for their high fibre content and protein levels, promoting a feeling of fullness and satisfaction. This can be particularly beneficial for managing hunger and preventing overeating.

4. Flexibility in Food Choices

Zero-point foods provide flexibility and variety in your food choices. This flexibility allows you to experiment with different ingredients, flavours, and cuisines, making the dietary journey more enjoyable and sustainable.

5. Long-term Health Benefits

Consistently incorporating zero-point foods into your diet can contribute to long-term health benefits. From supporting heart health to maintaining stable blood sugar levels, the nutritional content of these foods positively impacts various aspects of your well-being.

As you embark on this chapter's exploration, embrace the multifaceted benefits of zero-point foods. Beyond being a tool for weight management, these foods become your allies in crafting a diet that is rich in nutrients, flavours, and health advantages. Let the journey into the world of zero point foods unfold, guiding you towards a lifestyle where mindful eating and nourishment coexist harmoniously.

Chapter 2: Getting Started with Zero Point Cooking

Setting Up Your Zero Point Kitchen

Embarking on your journey into the world of Zero Point Cooking involves more than just following recipes; it's about creating an environment that supports your culinary exploration. In this chapter, we'll guide you through setting up your Zero Point Kitchen, from essential ingredients to must-have tools and the art of efficient meal planning and grocery shopping.

Essential Ingredients to Have on Hand

Fruits and Vegetables

Ensure your kitchen is stocked with a colourful array of fresh fruits and vegetables. These form the backbone of zero-point meals, offering essential vitamins, minerals, and fibre. From leafy greens to vibrant berries, having a variety on hand allows for endless creative possibilities.

Lean Proteins

Lean proteins are the building blocks of satisfying and nutritious meals. Keep options such as skinless poultry, lean cuts of meat, tofu, and legumes in your kitchen arsenal. These protein sources not only add depth to your dishes but also contribute to a feeling of fullness.

Whole Grains

Whole grains bring texture and substance to your meals. Brown rice, quinoa, whole wheat pasta, and oats are excellent choices. Incorporating these grains into your recipes provides a source of complex carbohydrates and additional nutritional benefits.

Greek Yogurt and Cottage Cheese

These dairy options are not only versatile but also rich in protein. Greek yoghurt and cottage cheese can be used in both sweet and savoury dishes, adding creaminess and a protein boost without the points.

Herbs and Spices

Elevate the flavours of your dishes without adding points by incorporating a variety of herbs and spices. From basil and oregano to cumin and turmeric, a well-stocked spice cabinet opens up a world of culinary possibilities.

Kitchen Tools and Equipment for Zero Point Cooking

Quality Knives and Cutting Boards

Invest in a set of sharp knives and durable cutting boards. Precise and efficient chopping not only speeds up your cooking process but also enhances the presentation of your dishes.

Non-Stick Cookware

Non-stick pans and pots are essential for cooking with minimal added fats. These kitchen workhorses make it easy to sauté, stir-fry, and cook proteins without worrying about excessive oil.

Food Scale and Measuring Cups

Accuracy in portion control is key to zero point cooking. A digital food scale and measuring cups help you portion ingredients accurately, ensuring your recipes stay on track.

Blender or Food Processor

These appliances are versatile tools for creating smooth sauces, dips, and soups. They are especially useful for incorporating zero-point vegetables into your recipes in a convenient and flavorful way.

Steamer Basket

Steaming is a healthy cooking method that preserves the nutritional worth of your ingredients. A steamer basket is perfect for cooking vegetables, fish, and even grains.

Meal Planning and Grocery Shopping

Creating Zero Point Meal Plans

Efficient meal planning is at the core of successful zero point cooking. Begin by identifying your favourite zero point foods and build your meals around them. Consider incorporating a variety of colours, textures, and flavours to keep your meals interesting.

- Breakfast: Plan energising meals with a mix of fruits, whole grains, and proteins.

- Lunch: Create satisfying salads, wraps, or hearty soups using a combination of lean proteins and fresh vegetables.

- Dinner: Explore diverse cuisines by incorporating different proteins, grains, and vegetables. One-pan meals or sheet pan dinners can simplify your cooking routine.

- Snacks: Prepare zero point snacks like fruit salads, yoghurt parfaits, or crunchy veggies with a flavorful dip.

Smart Grocery Shopping Tips for Zero Point Recipes

Navigating the grocery store strategically is the key to maintaining a well-stocked Zero Point Kitchen. Consider these tips:

- Plan Ahead: Create a list based on your meal plan to avoid impulsive purchases.

- Shop the Perimeter: The perimeter of the store often contains fresh produce, lean proteins, and dairy—essential components of zero point cooking.

- Read Labels: Even within the world of zero point foods, it's crucial to read labels for processed items. Be mindful of added sugars, preservatives, and unnecessary additives.

- Buy in Bulk: Purchase staple items like grains, legumes, and frozen fruits in bulk to save money in the long run.

- Explore the Frozen Aisle: Frozen vegetables and fruits can be just as nutritious as fresh ones and have a longer shelf life.

By embracing these foundational elements, you're not just setting up a kitchen; you're laying the groundwork for a sustainable and enjoyable Zero Point Cooking experience. The right ingredients and tools, coupled with thoughtful planning, will empower you to create delicious and nourishing meals without the worry of added points. Let the journey into your Zero Point Kitchen unfold, making every meal a delightful step towards your health and wellness goals.

Chapter 3: Frequently Asked Questions

Addressing Common Concerns

Can I Really Eat Unlimited Zero Point Foods?

One of the common questions that arise when delving into the world of zero point cooking is the notion of unlimited consumption. While zero point foods offer flexibility, it's crucial to strike a balance. The concept of "unlimited" doesn't imply an endless indulgence but rather an encouragement to prioritise these foods in your daily meals. Portion control remains vital even with zero point foods to ensure a well-rounded and balanced diet. Understanding your body's hunger and satiety cues becomes key in navigating the path of incorporating these foods in a mindful and health-conscious way.

How Do I Calculate Portion Sizes?

Calculating portion sizes is an integral aspect of successful zero point cooking. While these foods may carry zero points, portion control remains pivotal for effective weight management. Utilising measuring tools, such as a food scale and measuring cups, empowers you to gauge accurate serving sizes. It's essential to align portion sizes with your individual nutritional needs, taking into account factors like activity level, metabolism, and personal health goals. By being mindful of portions, you can enjoy zero point foods without compromising your overall dietary objectives.

Understanding Zero Point Food Labels

Decoding Nutrition Labels for Zero Point Items

Navigating nutrition labels is a skill that enhances your ability to make informed food choices. When it comes to zero point items, understanding the nutritional content is paramount. While these foods may be zero points, it's beneficial to examine labels for additional nutritional information, such as protein content, fibre, and potential additives. By decoding nutrition labels, you gain insight into the overall nutritional profile of the food, aiding you in creating a more balanced and varied diet.

Hidden Pitfalls to Watch Out For

Despite being zero points, certain pitfalls can lurk within food items. It's essential to be vigilant about added sugars, excessive sodium, or processed ingredients that may compromise the health benefits of these foods. Additionally, pre-packaged zero point items may contain hidden additives or preservatives. A discerning eye on labels ensures that your zero point choices contribute positively to your nutritional goals.

Customising Zero Point Recipes

Adjusting Flavours and Textures Without Adding Points

Customising zero point recipes allows you to tailor your meals to suit your taste preferences without compromising their point value. Experimenting with herbs, spices, and other flavour enhancers adds depth and variety to your dishes. Techniques like grilling, roasting, or sautéing can elevate textures and enhance the overall culinary experience. Understanding the art of flavour balance empowers you to create satisfying meals that align with your personal taste preferences.

Incorporating Personal Preferences and Dietary Restrictions

Zero point cooking is inherently versatile, allowing for the inclusion of personal preferences and accommodating dietary restrictions. Whether you follow a vegetarian, vegan, gluten-free, or any other specific dietary plan, zero point recipes can be adapted to suit your needs. Substituting ingredients, exploring alternative cooking methods, and embracing a variety of cuisines ensure that zero point cooking becomes a personalised and enjoyable journey.

By addressing these frequently asked questions, you gain a deeper understanding of the nuances involved in zero point cooking. From portion control to label scrutiny and customization, these insights empower you to navigate the world of zero point foods with confidence, making your culinary experience not only healthy but also uniquely yours.

Chapter 4: Ten (10) Delicious Zero Point Breakfast Recipes

1. Scrambled Eggs with Spinach and Tomatoes

Ingredients:
- 2 eggs
- 1 cup fresh spinach
- 1/2 cup cherry tomatoes, halved
- Salt and pepper to taste

Instructions:
1. Heat a non-stick pan over medium heat.
2. Add spinach and tomatoes to the pan and sauté until spinach wilts.
3. In a bowl, whisk eggs. Season with salt and pepper.
4. Pour eggs into the pan with vegetables and scramble until cooked.
5. Serve hot.

Nutritional Information:
Calories: ~250 kcal

Protein: ~20g
Fat: ~15g
Carbohydrates: ~10g

2. Greek Yogurt Parfait with Berries

Ingredients:
- 1 cup Greek yoghourt (unsweetened)
- 1/2 cup mixed berries (strawberries, blueberries, raspberries)
- 1 tablespoon honey
- Granola (optional)

Instructions:
1. In a glass, layer Greek yoghurt and mixed berries.
2. Drizzle honey over the top.
3. Add granola if desired.
4. Repeat layers.
5. Serve chilled.

Nutritional Information:
Calories: ~300 kcal
Protein: ~20g
Fat: ~10g
Carbohydrates: ~30g

3. Vegetable Omelette with Bell Peppers and Onions

Ingredients:
- 2 eggs

- 1/2 cup bell peppers, diced
- 1/4 cup onions, diced
- Salt and pepper to taste
- Olive oil for cooking

Instructions:

1. In a bowl, whisk eggs. Season with salt and pepper.
2. Heat olive oil in a pan over medium heat.
3. Add bell peppers and onions, sauté until softened.
4. Pour whisked eggs over vegetables, cook until set.
5. Fold omelette in half and serve.

Nutritional Information:

Calories: ~220 kcal

Protein: ~14g

Fat: ~15g

Carbohydrates: ~8g

4. Grilled Chicken Breast with Salsa

Ingredients:

- 1 boneless, skinless chicken breast
- 1/2 cup salsa
- 1 teaspoon olive oil
- Salt and pepper to taste

Instructions:

1. Preheat a grill or grill pan.
2. Brush the chicken breast with olive oil and season with salt and pepper.

3. Grill chicken until fully cooked.

4. Top with salsa before serving.

Nutritional Information:

Calories: ~200 kcal

Protein: ~25g

Fat: ~7g

Carbohydrates: ~10g

5. Overnight Oats with Chia Seeds and Fruit

Ingredients:
- 1/2 cup rolled oats
- 1/2 cup Greek yoghourt
- 1/2 cup milk (dairy or plant-based)
- 1 tablespoon chia seeds
- Mixed fruit for topping (e.g., berries, banana slices)

Instructions:

1. In a jar, combine oats, Greek yoghurt, milk, and chia seeds.

2. Stir well, cover, and refrigerate overnight.

3. In the morning, top with mixed fruit before serving.

Nutritional Information:

Calories: ~300 kcal

Protein: ~15g

Fat: ~10g

Carbohydrates: ~40g

6. Turkey and Veggie Breakfast Burrito (using lettuce as a wrap)

Ingredients:
- 4 large lettuce leaves
- 4 ounces cooked turkey, ground or sliced
- 1/2 cup bell peppers, diced
- 1/4 cup onions, diced
- Salsa for topping

Instructions:
1. Lay out lettuce leaves as wraps.
2. Fill each with turkey, bell peppers, and onions.
3. Top with salsa.
4. Roll up and serve.

Nutritional Information:
Calories: ~250 kcal
Protein: ~25g
Fat: ~10g
Carbohydrates: ~15g

7. Smoked Salmon and Cucumber Rolls

Ingredients:
- 4 ounces smoked salmon
- 1 cucumber, thinly sliced
- Cream cheese (optional)
- Fresh dill for garnish

Instructions:
1. Lay out cucumber slices.
2. Add a layer of smoked salmon on each slice.
3. Optionally, add a small amount of cream cheese.

4. Roll up and secure with a toothpick.
5. Garnish with fresh dill.

Nutritional Information:
  Calories: ~180 kcal
  Protein: ~20g
  Fat: ~10g
  Carbohydrates: ~5g

8. Black Bean and Corn Salad with Poached Egg

Ingredients:
  - 1 cup black beans (canned, drained and rinsed)
  - 1 cup corn kernels (fresh or frozen, cooked)
  - Cherry tomatoes, halved
  - 1 poached egg
  - Cilantro for garnish
  - Lime wedges

Instructions:
  1. In a bowl, combine black beans, corn, and cherry tomatoes.
  2. Top with a poached egg.
  3. Garnish with cilantro and serve with lime wedges.

Nutritional Information:
  Calories: ~300 kcal
  Protein: ~15g
  Fat: ~8g
  Carbohydrates: ~45g

9. Tofu Scramble with Mushrooms and Spinach

Ingredients:
- 1/2 cup firm tofu, crumbled
- 1/2 cup mushrooms, sliced
- 1 cup fresh spinach
- 1 clove garlic, minced
- Turmeric, salt, and pepper to taste

Instructions:
1. In a pan, sauté mushrooms and garlic until softened.
2. Add crumbled tofu and turmeric, stir well.
3. Add fresh spinach and cook until wilted.
4. Season with salt and pepper before serving.

Nutritional Information:
Calories: ~200 kcal
Protein: ~15g
Fat: ~12g
Carbohydrates: ~10g

10. Baked Cod with Lemon and Dill

Ingredients:
- 6 ounces cod fillet
- Lemon slices
- Fresh dill, chopped
- Salt and pepper to taste

Instructions:
1. Preheat the oven to 375°F (190°C).

2. Place cod on a baking sheet.
3. Season with salt and pepper, top with lemon slices and fresh dill.
4. Bake for 15-20 minutes or until the fish flakes easily.

Nutritional Information:

Calories: ~180 kcal

Protein: ~25g

Fat: ~8g

Carbohydrates: ~1g

Chapter 5: Ten (10) Savory Zero Point Lunch Recipes

1. Grilled Chicken Salad with Mixed Greens

Ingredients:
- 6 ounces grilled chicken breast, sliced
- Mixed salad greens (e.g., lettuce, spinach)
- Cherry tomatoes, halved
- Cucumber, sliced
- Red onion, thinly sliced
- Balsamic vinaigrette dressing

Instructions:
1. Arrange mixed greens on a plate.
2. Top with grilled chicken, cherry tomatoes, cucumber, and red onion.
3. Drizzle with balsamic vinaigrette dressing.

Nutritional Information:

Calories: ~300 kcal
Protein: ~30g
Fat: ~10g
Carbohydrates: ~20g

2. Vegetable Stir-Fry with Tofu

Ingredients:
- 1 cup tofu, cubed
- Mixed stir-fry vegetables (e.g., snap peas, bell peppers, broccoli)
- Soy sauce
- Sesame oil
- Ginger and garlic, minced

Instructions:
1. In a wok or pan, stir-fry tofu until golden.
2. Add mixed vegetables, ginger, and garlic.
3. Stir in soy sauce and sesame oil.
4. Cook until vegetables are tender.

Nutritional Information:
Calories: ~250 kcal
Protein: ~15g
Fat: ~15g
Carbohydrates: ~20g

3. Shrimp and Zucchini Noodles

Ingredients:
- 6 ounces shrimp, peeled and deveined
- Zucchini noodles

- Cherry tomatoes, halved
- Olive oil
- Lemon juice
- Fresh parsley for garnish

Instructions:
1. Sauté shrimp in olive oil until cooked.
2. Add zucchini noodles and cherry tomatoes, cook until tender.
3. Drizzle with lemon juice and garnish with fresh parsley.

Nutritional Information:
Calories: ~200 kcal
Protein: ~25g
Fat: ~10g
Carbohydrates: ~10g

4. Lentil Soup with Vegetables

Ingredients:
- 1 cup dry lentils
- Carrots, celery, and onions, diced
- Vegetable broth
- Garlic, minced
- Cumin and paprika
- Salt and pepper to taste

Instructions:
1. Rinse lentils and cook in vegetable broth until tender.
2. Sauté garlic, carrots, celery, and onions in a pot.
3. Add cooked lentils, cumin, paprika, salt, and pepper.
4. Simmer until vegetables are cooked.

Nutritional Information:
  Calories: ~250 kcal
  Protein: ~15g
  Fat: ~1g
  Carbohydrates: ~45g

5. Turkey Lettuce Wraps with Avocado

Ingredients:
  - 8 ounces ground turkey
  - Lettuce leaves (e.g., iceberg or butter lettuce)
  - Avocado, sliced
  - Tomatoes, diced
  - Cilantro for garnish
  - Salsa (optional)

Instructions:
  1. Cook ground turkey until browned.
  2. Arrange lettuce leaves on a plate.
  3. Fill with turkey, avocado, and tomatoes.
  4. Garnish with cilantro and serve with salsa if desired.

Nutritional Information:
  Calories: ~300 kcal
  Protein: ~25g
  Fat: ~15g
  Carbohydrates: ~20g

6. Quinoa Salad with Chickpeas and Veggies

Ingredients:

- 1 cup cooked quinoa
- Chickpeas (canned, drained and rinsed)
- Cherry tomatoes, halved
- Cucumber, diced
- Red bell pepper, diced
- Feta cheese (optional)
- Olive oil and lemon dressing

Instructions:
1. In a bowl, combine quinoa, chickpeas, tomatoes, cucumber, and bell pepper.
2. Add feta cheese if desired.
3. Drizzle with olive oil and lemon dressing.

Nutritional Information:
Calories: ~350 kcal
Protein: ~15g
Fat: ~15g
Carbohydrates: ~40g

7. Baked Salmon with Lemon and Asparagus

Ingredients:
- 6 ounces salmon fillet
- Asparagus spears
- Lemon slices
- Olive oil
- Garlic powder, salt, and pepper

Instructions:

1. Preheat the oven to 400°F (200°C).
2. Place salmon on a baking sheet, surrounded with asparagus.
3. Drizzle olive oil over salmon and asparagus.
4. Season with garlic powder, salt, and pepper.
5. Top with lemon slices.
6. Bake for 15-20 minutes until the salmon is done.

Nutritional Information:
Calories: ~300 kcal
Protein: ~25g
Fat: ~20g
Carbohydrates: ~5g

8. Egg Salad Lettuce Wraps

Ingredients:
- 4 hard-boiled eggs, chopped
- Greek yoghourt
- Dijon mustard
- Green onions, chopped
- Lettuce leaves for wrapping

Instructions:
1. In a bowl, mix chopped eggs, Greek yoghurt, mustard, and green onions.
2. Spoon egg salad on lettuce leaves.
3. Roll up and serve.

Nutritional Information:
Calories: ~200 kcal
Protein: ~15g

Fat: ~12g
Carbohydrates: ~5g

9. Black Bean and Vegetable Burrito Bowl

Ingredients:
- 1 cup black beans (canned, drained and rinsed)
- Brown rice, cooked
- Bell peppers, diced
- Corn kernels (fresh or frozen, cooked)
- Salsa
- Avocado slices

Instructions:
1. In a bowl, layer black beans, brown rice, bell peppers, and corn.
2. Top with salsa and avocado slices.

Nutritional Information:
Calories: ~300 kcal
Protein: ~15g
Fat: ~10g
Carbohydrates: ~45g

10. Cabbage and Carrot Slaw with Grilled Chicken

Ingredients:
- 6 ounces grilled chicken breast, shredded
- Green cabbage, thinly sliced
- Carrots, grated
- Greek yoghourt dressing
- Cilantro for garnish

Instructions:

1. In a bowl, combine shredded chicken, cabbage, and carrots.
2. Toss with Greek yoghurt dressing.
3. Garnish with cilantro.

Nutritional Information:

Calories: ~250 kcal

Protein: ~25g

Fat: ~10g

Carbohydrates: ~15g

Chapter 6: Ten (10) Delectable Zero Point Dinner Recipes

1. Grilled Salmon with Lemon and Dill

Ingredients:
- 6 ounces salmon fillet
- Lemon slices
- Fresh dill
- Olive oil
- Salt and pepper

Instructions:
1. Preheat the grill.
2. Place the salmon on a piece of foil.
3. Drizzle with olive oil, season with salt and pepper.
4. Top with lemon slices and fresh dill.
5. Grill for 10-15 minutes until the salmon is done.

Nutritional Information:

Calories: ~300 kcal
Protein: ~25g
Fat: ~20g
Carbohydrates: ~2g

2. Chicken and Vegetable Stir-Fry

Ingredients:
- 8 ounces boneless, skinless chicken breast, sliced
- Mixed stir-fry vegetables (e.g., snap peas, bell peppers, broccoli)
- Soy sauce
- Sesame oil
- Garlic and ginger, minced

Instructions:
1. In a wok or pan, stir-fry chicken until cooked.
2. Add mixed vegetables, garlic, and ginger.
3. Stir in soy sauce and sesame oil.
4. Cook until vegetables are tender.

Nutritional Information:
Calories: ~250 kcal
Protein: ~25g
Fat: ~10g
Carbohydrates: ~15g

3. Baked Cod with Herbs and Tomatoes

Ingredients:
- 6 ounces cod fillet
- Cherry tomatoes, halved

- Fresh herbs (e.g., parsley, thyme)
- Olive oil
- Garlic, minced
- Lemon juice

Instructions:

1. Preheat the oven to 375°F (190°C).
2. Place cod on a baking sheet.
3. Surround with cherry tomatoes and minced garlic.
4. Drizzle with olive oil and lemon juice.
5. Bake for 15-20 minutes or until the cod is cooked.

Nutritional Information:

Calories: ~200 kcal
Protein: ~25g
Fat: ~10g
Carbohydrates: ~5g

4. Vegetable and Chickpea Curry

Ingredients:

- Chickpeas (canned, drained and rinsed)
- Mixed vegetables (e.g., carrots, peas, cauliflower)
- Coconut milk
- Curry powder
- Onion and garlic, minced
- Fresh cilantro for garnish

Instructions:

1. In a pot, sauté onion and garlic until softened.
2. Add mixed vegetables, chickpeas, and curry powder.

3. Pour in coconut milk and simmer until vegetables are cooked.
4. Garnish with fresh cilantro.

Nutritional Information:
  Calories: ~300 kcal
  Protein: ~15g
  Fat: ~15g
  Carbohydrates: ~35g

5. Zucchini Noodles with Pesto and Cherry Tomatoes

Ingredients:
  - Zucchini noodles
  - Cherry tomatoes, halved
  - Pesto sauce
  - Parmesan cheese (optional)
  - Pine nuts for garnish

Instructions:
  1. In a pan, sauté zucchini noodles until tender.
  2. Add cherry tomatoes and heat through.
  3. Toss with pesto sauce.
  4. Garnish with Parmesan cheese and pine nuts.

Nutritional Information:
  Calories: ~250 kcal
  Protein: ~8g
  Fat: ~20g
  Carbohydrates: ~10g

6. Turkey and Quinoa Stuffed Bell Peppers

Ingredients:
- Bell peppers, halved
- Ground turkey
- Cooked quinoa
- Black beans (canned, drained and rinsed)
- Salsa
- Mexican blend cheese (optional)

Instructions:
1. Preheat the oven to 375°F (190°C).
2. In a bowl, mix ground turkey, cooked quinoa, black beans, and salsa.
3. Stuff bell peppers with the mixture.
4. Top with cheese if desired.
5. Bake for 25-30 minutes or until peppers are tender.

Nutritional Information:
Calories: ~350 kcal
Protein: ~25g
Fat: ~15g
Carbohydrates: ~30g

7. Shrimp and Broccoli Skewers

Ingredients:
- Shrimp, peeled and deveined
- Broccoli florets
- Olive oil
- Lemon zest and juice
- Garlic, minced
- Paprika and black pepper

Instructions:
1. Preheat the grill or oven.
2. Thread shrimp and broccoli onto skewers.
3. Mix olive oil, lemon zest, lemon juice, garlic, paprika, and black pepper.
4. Brush skewers with the mixture.
5. Grill or bake for 8-10 minutes, until the prawns are opaque.

Nutritional Information:
Calories: ~200 kcal
Protein: ~25g
Fat: ~10g
Carbohydrates: ~8g

8. Eggplant and Tomato Bake

Ingredients:
- Eggplant, sliced
- Cherry tomatoes, halved
- Mozzarella cheese, shredded
- Fresh basil leaves
- Olive oil
- Balsamic glaze (optional)

Instructions:
1. Preheat the oven to 375°F (190°C).
2. Arrange eggplant slices on a baking sheet.
3. Top with cherry tomatoes and mozzarella cheese.
4. Drizzle with olive oil.
5. Bake for 20-25 minutes, or until the cheese melts and bubbles.
6. Garnish with fresh basil and drizzle with balsamic glaze if desired.

Nutritional Information:
Calories: ~250 kcal
Protein: ~10g
Fat: ~15g
Carbohydrates: ~20g

9. Spinach and Mushroom Stuffed Chicken Breast

Ingredients:
- Chicken breast
- Spinach, wilted
- Mushrooms, sliced and sautéed
- Feta cheese
- Olive oil
- Italian seasoning

Instructions:
1. Preheat the oven to 375°F (190°C).
2. Cut a pocket into each chicken breast.
3. Stuff with wilted spinach, sautéed mushrooms, and feta cheese.
4. Rub with olive oil and sprinkle with Italian seasoning.
5. Bake for 25-30 minutes, or until the chicken is cooked thoroughly.

Nutritional Information:
Calories: ~300 kcal
Protein: ~30g
Fat: ~15g
Carbohydrates: ~5g

10. Cauliflower Fried Rice with Tofu

Ingredients:
- Cauliflower rice
- Extra-firm tofu, cubed
- Mixed vegetables (e.g., peas, carrots, corn)
- Soy sauce
- Sesame oil
- Green onions, chopped

Instructions:
1. In a pan, sauté tofu until golden.
2. Add mixed vegetables and cauliflower rice.
3. Stir in soy sauce and sesame oil.
4. Cook until vegetables are tender.
5. Garnish with chopped green onions.

Nutritional Information:
Calories: ~250 kcal
Protein: ~15g
Fat: ~15g
Carbohydrates: ~20g

Chapter 7: Ten (10) Irresistible Zero Point Desserts Recipes

1. Mixed Berry Salad

Ingredients:
- Mixed berries (e.g., strawberries, blueberries, raspberries)
- Fresh mint leaves
- Lemon juice

Instructions:
1. Wash and prepare the berries.
2. Toss them together in a bowl.
3. Drizzle with fresh lemon juice.
4. Garnish with mint leaves.

Nutritional Information:
Calories: ~50 kcal
Protein: ~1g
Fat: ~0.5g

Carbohydrates: ~12g

2. Grilled Pineapple with Cinnamon

Ingredients:
- Pineapple slices
- Ground cinnamon

Instructions:
1. Preheat the grill or grill pan.
2. Grill pineapple slices for a few minutes on each side.
3. Sprinkle it with ground cinnamon before serving.

Nutritional Information:
Calories: ~60 kcal
Protein: ~0.5g
Fat: ~0.2g
Carbohydrates: ~16g

3. Baked Apples with Cinnamon

Ingredients:
- Apples, cored and sliced
- Ground cinnamon
- Stevia or sweetener of choice

Instructions:
1. Preheat the oven to 375°F (190°C).
2. Place apple slices in a baking dish.
3. Sprinkle it with cinnamon and sweetener.
4. Bake for 20-25 minutes or until the apples are tender.

Nutritional Information:
    Calories: ~80 kcal
    Protein: ~0.5g
    Fat: ~0.3g
    Carbohydrates: ~22g

4. Sugar-Free Jello with Fruit

Ingredients:
    - Sugar-free gelatin
    - Mixed fruit (e.g., berries, orange segments)

Instructions:
    1. Prepare sugar-free gelatin according to package instructions.
    2. Once it starts to set, fold in mixed fruit.
    3. Refrigerate until fully set.

Nutritional Information:
    Calories: ~10 kcal (for sugar-free gelatin)
    Protein: ~1g
    Fat: ~0g
    Carbohydrates: ~2g

5. Watermelon and Mint Salad

Ingredients:
    - Watermelon, cubed
    - Fresh mint leaves
    - Lime juice

Instructions:

1. Mix watermelon cubes in a bowl.
2. Toss with fresh mint leaves.
3. Drizzle with lime juice.

Nutritional Information:
    Calories: ~40 kcal
    Protein: ~1g
    Fat: ~0g
    Carbohydrates: ~10g

6. Berry Frozen Yogurt Bites

Ingredients:
    - Greek yoghourt
    - Mixed berries (e.g., blueberries, raspberries)

Instructions:
    1. Mix Greek yoghurt with berries.
    2. Spoon small portions onto a baking sheet.
    3. Freeze until solid.

Nutritional Information:
    Calories: ~30 kcal
    Protein: ~2g
    Fat: ~0g
    Carbohydrates: ~5g

7. Cucumber Mint Sorbet

Ingredients:
    - Cucumber, peeled and diced

- Fresh mint leaves
- Lemon juice
- Stevia or sweetener of choice

Instructions:
1. Blend cucumber, mint, lemon juice, and sweetener until smooth.
2. Pour into a container and freeze until firm.

Nutritional Information:
Calories: ~20 kcal
Protein: ~1g
Fat: ~0g
Carbohydrates: ~5g

8. Sugar-Free Gelatin Cups

Ingredients:
- Sugar-free gelatin
- Fresh fruit for garnish (e.g., berries)

Instructions:
1. Prepare sugar-free gelatin according to package instructions.
2. Pour into individual cups.
3. Refrigerate until fully set.
4. Garnish with fresh fruit before serving.

Nutritional Information:
Calories: ~10 kcal (for sugar-free gelatin)
Protein: ~1g
Fat: ~0g
Carbohydrates: ~2g

9. Orange Slices with Tajin

Ingredients:
  - Orange slices
  - Tajin seasoning

Instructions:
  1. Slice oranges into wedges.
  2. Sprinkle Tajin seasoning over the slices.

Nutritional Information:
  Calories: ~40 kcal
  Protein: ~1g
  Fat: ~0g
  Carbohydrates: ~9g

10. Kiwi and Strawberry Skewers

Ingredients:
  - Kiwi, peeled and sliced
  - Strawberries, hulled
  - Wooden skewers

Instructions:
  1. Alternate threading kiwi slices and strawberries onto skewers.
  2. Chill in the refrigerator before serving.

Nutritional Information:
  Calories: ~30 kcal
  Protein: ~1g
  Fat: ~0g

Carbohydrates: ~7g

Chapter 8: Ten (10) Sweet Zero Point Sides and Snacks

1. Sliced Cucumber with Hummus

Ingredients:
- Cucumber, sliced
- Hummus

Instructions:
   1. Slice the cucumber into rounds.
   2. Serve with hummus for dipping.

Nutritional Information:
   Calories: ~50 kcal
   Protein: ~2g
   Fat: ~3g
   Carbohydrates: ~7g

2. Roasted Brussels Sprouts

Ingredients:
- Brussels sprouts, trimmed and halved
- Olive oil
- Salt and pepper

Instructions:
1. Preheat the oven to 400°F (200°C).
2. Toss Brussels sprouts with olive oil, salt, and pepper.
3. Roast for 20-25 minutes or until crispy.

Nutritional Information:
Calories: ~50 kcal
Protein: ~2g
Fat: ~3g
Carbohydrates: ~8g

3. Jicama Sticks with Lime and Chili Powder

Ingredients:
- Jicama, peeled and cut into sticks
- Lime juice
- Chili powder

Instructions:
1. Peel and cut jicama into sticks.
2. Drizzle with lime juice and sprinkle with chilli powder.

Nutritional Information:
Calories: ~30 kcal
Protein: ~1g
Fat: ~0g

Carbohydrates: ~8g

4. Pickles or Pickled Vegetables

Ingredients:
- Pickles or assorted pickled vegetables

Instructions:
1. Simply serve pickles or pickled vegetables as a snack.

Nutritional Information:
Calories: ~10 kcal (per pickle, actual values may vary)
Protein: ~0g
Fat: ~0g
Carbohydrates: ~2g

5. Air-Popped Popcorn

Ingredients:
- Popcorn kernels

Instructions:
1. Pop the popcorn using an air popper.
2. Season with a sprinkle of salt or other desired seasonings.

Nutritional Information:
Calories: ~30 kcal (for 1 cup, air-popped)
Protein: ~1g
Fat: ~0g
Carbohydrates: ~6g

6. Celery Sticks with Peanut Butter

Ingredients:
- Celery sticks
- Peanut butter

Instructions:
1. Cut celery into sticks.
2. Spread peanut butter on the celery.

Nutritional Information:
Calories: ~50 kcal
Protein: ~2g
Fat: ~4g
Carbohydrates: ~3g

7. Steamed Edamame

Ingredients:
- Edamame in the pod
- Sea salt (optional)

Instructions:
1. Steam edamame until tender.
2. Sprinkle with sea salt if desired.

Nutritional Information:
Calories: ~100 kcal (for 1 cup)
Protein: ~8g
Fat: ~4g
Carbohydrates: ~8g

8. Cherry Tomatoes with Balsamic Glaze

Ingredients:
- Cherry tomatoes
- Balsamic glaze

Instructions:
1. Wash and halve cherry tomatoes.
2. Drizzle with balsamic glaze.

Nutritional Information:
Calories: ~30 kcal
Protein: ~1g
Fat: ~0g
Carbohydrates: ~7g

9. Radish Slices with Sea Salt

Ingredients:
- Radishes, thinly sliced
- Sea salt

Instructions:
1. Slice radishes into thin rounds.
2. Sprinkle it with sea salt.

Nutritional Information:
Calories: ~15 kcal
Protein: ~1g
Fat: ~0g
Carbohydrates: ~3g

10. Seaweed Snacks

Ingredients:
- Seaweed snack sheets

Instructions:
1. Simply enjoy seaweed snack sheets as a light, crispy snack.

Nutritional Information:
Calories: ~10 kcal (per sheet, actual values may vary)
Protein: ~1g
Fat: ~0g
Carbohydrates: ~1g

Chapter 9: Ten (10) Nourishing Zero Point Beverages

1. Water

Ingredients:
- Water

Instructions:
1. Pour water into a glass or bottle.
2. Serve chilled or at room temperature.

Nutritional Information:
Calories: 0 kcal
Protein: 0g
Fat: 0g
Carbohydrates: 0g

2. Black Coffee (without additives)

Ingredients:
- Coffee grounds or beans
- Water

Instructions:
1. Brew black coffee using your preferred method.
2. Serve hot.

Nutritional Information:
Calories: ~2 kcal (for 8 oz)
Protein: 0g
Fat: 0g
Carbohydrates: 0g

3. Herbal Tea (without sugar)

Ingredients:
- Herbal tea bag or loose leaves
- Water

Instructions:
1. Steep the herbal tea bag or leaves in hot water.
2. Let it steep for a few minutes.
3. Remove the tea bag, or sieve the leaves.
4. Serve hot.

Nutritional Information:
Calories: 0 kcal
Protein: 0g
Fat: 0g
Carbohydrates: 0g

4. Green Tea (without sugar)

Ingredients:
- Green tea bag or loose leaves
- Water

Instructions:
1. Steep the green tea bag or leaves in hot water.
2. Let it steep for a few minutes.
3. Remove the tea bag, or sieve the leaves.
4. Serve hot.

Nutritional Information:
Calories: 0 kcal
Protein: 0g
Fat: 0g
Carbohydrates: 0g

5. Sparkling Water (plain)

Ingredients:
- Plain sparkling water

Instructions:
1. Pour plain sparkling water into a glass or serve directly from the bottle.
2. Serve chilled.

Nutritional Information:
Calories: 0 kcal
Protein: 0g

Fat: 0g
Carbohydrates: 0g

6. Iced Coffee (black, without sugar)

Ingredients:
- Coffee grounds or beans
- Water
- Ice cubes

Instructions:
1. Brew black coffee using your preferred method.
2. Allow the coffee to cool.
3. Pour the cooled coffee over ice cubes.
4. Serve chilled.

Nutritional Information:
Calories: ~2 kcal (for 8 oz)
Protein: 0g
Fat: 0g
Carbohydrates: 0g

7. Unsweetened Almond Milk

Ingredients:
- Unsweetened almond milk

Instructions:
1. Pour unsweetened almond milk into a glass.
2. Serve chilled.

Nutritional Information:
  Calories: ~13 kcal (for 1 cup)
  Protein: ~1g
  Fat: ~1g
  Carbohydrates: ~0.5g

8. Diet Soda

Ingredients:
  - Diet soda of your choice

Instructions:
  1. Pour diet soda into a glass or serve directly from the can or bottle.
  2. Serve chilled.

Nutritional Information:
  Calories: 0 kcal
  Protein: 0g
  Fat: 0g
  Carbohydrates: 0g

9. Hot Lemon Water

Ingredients:
  - Fresh lemon
  - Water

Instructions:
  1. Squeeze fresh lemon juice into hot water.
  2. Optionally, add a slice of lemon.
  3. Serve hot.

Nutritional Information:
Calories: ~6 kcal (for 1 lemon)
Protein: 0g
Fat: 0g
Carbohydrates: ~2g

10. Black or Green Iced Tea (without sugar)

Ingredients:
- Black or green tea bag or loose leaves
- Water
- Ice cubes

Instructions:
1. Steep the tea bag or leaves in hot water.
2. Let it steep for a few minutes.
3. Remove the tea bag, or sieve the leaves.
4. Allow the tea to cool, then pour over ice cubes.
5. Serve chilled.

Nutritional Information:
Calories: 0 kcal
Protein: 0g
Fat: 0g
Carbohydrates: 0g

14 Day Meal Plan

Day 1

Breakfast:
Scrambled Eggs with Spinach and Tomatoes
- **Ingredients**: Eggs, spinach, tomatoes
- **Instructions**: Cook eggs with spinach and tomatoes until scrambled.

Lunch:
Grilled Chicken Salad with Mixed Greens
- **Ingredients**: Chicken breast, mixed greens, olive oil, lemon
- **Instructions**: Grill chicken, toss with mixed greens, and drizzle with olive oil and lemon.

Dinner:
Grilled Salmon with Lemon and Dill
- **Ingredients**: Salmon fillet, lemon, fresh dill
- **Instructions**: Grill salmon and top with lemon slices and fresh dill.

Day 2

Breakfast:
Greek Yogurt Parfait with Berries
- **Ingredients**: Greek yoghourt, berries
- **Instructions**: Layer Greek yoghurt with fresh berries.

Lunch:

Vegetable Omelette with Bell Peppers and Onions
- **Ingredients**: Eggs, bell peppers, onions
- **Instructions**: Make an omelette with bell peppers and onions.

Dinner:

Chicken and Vegetable Stir-Fry
- **Ingredients**: Chicken breast, mixed vegetables, soy sauce
- **Instructions**: Stir-fry chicken and vegetables with soy sauce.

Day 3

Breakfast:

Overnight Oats with Chia Seeds and Fruit
- **Ingredients**: Oats, chia seeds, fruit, almond milk
- **Instructions**: Mix oats, chia seeds, and almond milk. Refrigerate overnight, top with fruit.

Lunch:

Grilled Chicken Breast with Salsa
- **Ingredients**: Chicken breast, salsa
- **Instructions**: Grill chicken and top with salsa.

Dinner:

Baked Cod with Herbs and Tomatoes
- **Ingredients**: Cod fillet, cherry tomatoes, fresh herbs
- **Instructions**: Bake cod with tomatoes and herbs.

Day 4

Breakfast:

Turkey and Veggie Breakfast Burrito (using lettuce as a wrap)
- **Ingredients**: Ground turkey, lettuce, bell peppers, onions
- **Instructions**: Cook turkey with veggies, wrap in lettuce.

Lunch:

Black Bean and Corn Salad with Poached Egg
- **Ingredients**: Black beans, corn, poached egg
- **Instructions**: Toss black beans and corn, top with poached egg.

Dinner:

Turkey and Quinoa Stuffed Bell Peppers
- **Ingredients**: Ground turkey, quinoa, bell peppers
- **Instructions**: Stuff peppers with turkey and quinoa mixture, bake.

Day 5

Breakfast:

Tofu Scramble with Mushrooms and Spinach
- **Ingredients**: Tofu, mushrooms, spinach
- **Instructions**: Scramble tofu with mushrooms and spinach.

Lunch:

Baked Salmon with Lemon and Asparagus
- **Ingredients**: Salmon fillet, asparagus, lemon
- **Instructions**: Bake salmon with asparagus and lemon.

Dinner:

Vegetable and Chickpea Curry

- **Ingredients**: Chickpeas, mixed vegetables, coconut milk, curry powder
- **Instructions**: Cook chickpeas and veggies in coconut milk with curry powder.

Day 6

Breakfast:

Scrambled Eggs with Spinach and Tomatoes

- **Ingredients**: Eggs, spinach, tomatoes
- **Instructions**: Cook eggs with spinach and tomatoes until scrambled.

Lunch:

Quinoa Salad with Chickpeas and Veggies

- **Ingredients**: Quinoa, chickpeas, mixed vegetables
- **Instructions**: Toss cooked quinoa with chickpeas and veggies.

Dinner:

Zucchini Noodles with Pesto and Cherry Tomatoes

- **Ingredients**: Zucchini noodles, pesto, cherry tomatoes
- **Instructions**: Sauté zucchini noodles, toss with pesto and cherry tomatoes.

Day 7

Breakfast:

Greek Yogurt Parfait with Berries
- **Ingredients**: Greek yoghourt, berries
- **Instructions**: Layer Greek yoghurt with fresh berries.

Lunch:

Lentil Soup with Vegetables
- **Ingredients**: Lentils, mixed vegetables, broth
- **Instructions**: Cook lentils and veggies in broth.

Dinner:

Spinach and Mushroom Stuffed Chicken Breast
- **Ingredients**: Chicken breast, spinach, mushrooms
- **Instructions**: Stuff chicken with spinach and mushrooms, bake.

Day 8

Breakfast:

Overnight Oats with Chia Seeds and Fruit
- **Ingredients**: Oats, chia seeds, fruit, almond milk
- **Instructions**: Mix oats, chia seeds, and almond milk. Refrigerate overnight, top with fruit.

Lunch:

Turkey Lettuce Wraps with Avocado
- **Ingredients**: Ground turkey, lettuce, avocado

- **Instructions**: Cook turkey, wrap in lettuce, and top with avocado.

Dinner:
Cauliflower Fried Rice with Tofu
- **Ingredients**: Cauliflower rice, tofu, mixed vegetables
- **Instructions**: Sauté tofu and veggies, stir in cauliflower rice.

Day 9

Breakfast:
Scrambled Eggs with Spinach and Tomatoes
- **Ingredients**: Eggs, spinach, tomatoes
- **Instructions**: Cook eggs with spinach and tomatoes until scrambled.

Lunch:
Baked Cod with Lemon and Dill
- **Ingredients**: Cod fillet, lemon, fresh dill
- **Instructions**: Bake cod with lemon and dill.

Dinner:
Baked Salmon with Lemon and Asparagus
- **Ingredients**: Salmon fillet, asparagus, lemon
- **Instructions**: Bake salmon with asparagus and lemon.

Day 10

Breakfast:
Tofu Scramble with Mushrooms and Spinach
- **Ingredients**: Tofu, mushrooms, spinach
- **Instructions**: Scramble tofu with mushrooms and spinach.

Lunch:
Vegetable Stir-Fry with Tofu
- **Ingredients**: Tofu, mixed vegetables, soy sauce
- **Instructions**: Stir-fry tofu and vegetables with soy sauce.

Dinner:
Chicken and Vegetable Stir-Fry
- **Ingredients**: Chicken breast, mixed vegetables, soy sauce
- **Instructions**: Stir-fry chicken and vegetables with soy sauce.

Day 11

Breakfast:
Turkey and Veggie Breakfast Burrito (using lettuce as a wrap)
- **Ingredients**: Ground turkey, lettuce, bell peppers, onions
- **Instructions**: Cook turkey with veggies, wrap in lettuce.

Lunch:
Grilled Chicken Salad with Mixed Greens
- **Ingredients**: Chicken breast, mixed greens, olive oil, lemon
- **Instructions**: Grill chicken, toss with mixed greens, and drizzle

with olive oil and lemon.

Dinner:

Zucchini Noodles with Pesto and Cherry Tomatoes
- **Ingredients**: Zucchini noodles, pesto, cherry tomatoes
- **Instructions**: Sauté zucchini noodles, toss with pesto and cherry tomatoes.

Day 12

Breakfast:

Greek Yogurt Parfait with Berries
- **Ingredients**: Greek yoghourt, berries
- **Instructions**: Layer Greek yoghurt with fresh berries.

Lunch:

Black Bean and Vegetable Burrito Bowl
- **Ingredients**: Black beans, mixed vegetables, salsa
- **Instructions**: Combine black beans and veggies, top with salsa.

Dinner:

Turkey and Quinoa Stuffed Bell Peppers
- **Ingredients**: Ground turkey, quinoa, bell peppers
- **Instructions**: Stuff peppers with turkey and quinoa mixture, bake.

Day 13

Breakfast:

Overnight Oats with Chia Seeds and Fruit
- **Ingredients**: Oats, chia seeds, fruit, almond milk
- **Instructions**: Mix oats, chia seeds, and almond milk. Refrigerate overnight, top with fruit.

Lunch:

Egg Salad Lettuce Wraps
- **Ingredients**: Hard-boiled eggs, lettuce
- **Instructions**: Make egg salad, wrap in lettuce.

Dinner:

Shrimp and Zucchini Noodles
- **Ingredients**: Shrimp, zucchini noodles, garlic, olive oil
- **Instructions**: Sauté shrimp and zucchini noodles in garlic and olive oil.

Day 14

Breakfast:

Scrambled Eggs with Spinach and Tomatoes
- **Ingredients**: Eggs, spinach, tomatoes
- **Instructions**: Cook eggs with spinach and tomatoes until scrambled.

Lunch:

Cabbage and Carrot Slaw with Grilled Chicken
- **Ingredients**: Shredded cabbage and carrots, grilled chicken
- **Instructions**: Toss shredded vegetables, top with grilled chicken.

Dinner:
Vegetable and Chickpea Curry
- **Ingredients**: Chickpeas, mixed vegetables, coconut milk, curry powder
- **Instructions**: Cook chickpeas and veggies in coconut milk with curry powder.

11

Conclusion

As you reach the conclusion of this Zero Point Cookbook, you've embarked on a culinary journey that extends beyond the realm of recipes. Embracing the Zero Point Lifestyle is not just about what you eat; it's a holistic approach to wellness, celebrating successes, staying motivated, and cultivating a harmonious relationship with food.

Embracing the Zero Point Lifestyle

The Zero Point Lifestyle is more than a set of dietary guidelines; it's a mindset shift towards mindful and balanced living. Embracing this lifestyle involves viewing food as a source of nourishment and enjoyment, free from the constraints of rigid dieting. It's a commitment to making choices that align with your health goals while savouring the flavours and textures that make each meal a gratifying experience.

Celebrating Successes and Staying Motivated

Every step in your Zero Point Cooking journey is a success worth celebrating. Whether you've mastered a new recipe, achieved a personal wellness milestone, or simply found joy in the process of cooking, take a moment to acknowledge and celebrate these victories. The path to a healthier lifestyle is a series of small triumphs, and each one contributes to the mosaic of your overall well-being.

Staying motivated on this journey involves finding inspiration in various forms. Experimenting with new ingredients, exploring diverse cuisines, or sharing your experiences with a supportive community can rekindle your passion for a zero point lifestyle. Set realistic goals, track your progress, and allow each accomplishment to fuel your commitment to long-term health.

Long-term Strategies to Maintain a Healthy Relationship with Food

The Zero Point Lifestyle is not a short-term fix but a sustainable and enduring commitment to your well-being. To maintain a healthy relationship with food in the long term, consider the following strategies:

1. Variety is Key

Continue to explore the rich tapestry of flavours and ingredients that zero point cooking offers. The more variety you introduce into your meals, the more sustainable and enjoyable your dietary habits become.

2. Mindful Eating Practices

Practise mindful eating by savouring each bite, paying attention to hunger and fullness cues, and avoiding distractions during meals. This approach fosters a deeper connection with your food and encourages a more intuitive approach to eating.

3. Flexibility and Adaptability

Life is dynamic, and your dietary choices should be adaptable. Embrace the flexibility of the Zero Point Lifestyle by adjusting your meals to suit changing circumstances, occasions, or personal preferences.

4. Regular Physical Activity

Combine your zero point lifestyle with regular physical activity to promote overall health. Find activities that bring you joy, whether it's walking, jogging, yoga, or any other form of exercise.

5. Community and Support

Engage with a community of like-minded individuals who share similar health and wellness goals. Whether online or in-person, a supportive community provides encouragement, inspiration, and a platform to share experiences.

6. Continuous Learning

Stay informed about nutrition, wellness, and new culinary trends. The more you learn about the impact of food on your body and mind, the better equipped you are to make informed choices that align with your health goals.

7. Cultivate a Positive Mindset

Approach your Zero Point Lifestyle with a positive and compassionate mindset. Understand that the journey may have its ups and downs, but each day presents an opportunity to make choices that contribute to your well-being.

In concluding this cookbook, remember that the Zero Point Lifestyle is not a destination but a continuous, evolving journey. By celebrating successes, staying motivated, and embracing long-term strategies, you've laid the groundwork for a healthier and more fulfilling relationship with food. As you carry the principles of zero point cooking into your daily life, may each meal be a testament to the joy of nourishing your body, savouring the flavours, and embracing a lifestyle that supports your overall health and happiness. Cheers to your Zero Point Lifestyle!

12

Dear Reader,

Thank You for Embarking on Your Zero Point Journey

As you close the pages of this Zero Point Cookbook, I extend my heartfelt gratitude for joining this culinary exploration. Your commitment to embracing the Zero Point Lifestyle is a testament to your dedication to health, flavour, and the joy of mindful eating.

In the world of zeros and points, you've discovered a pathway that transcends mere recipes. It's a lifestyle that celebrates successes, finds motivation in each step, and fosters a lasting relationship with food. Your journey has been a mosaic of flavours, textures, and personal triumphs.

Thank you for allowing this cookbook to be a companion on your quest for wellness. May each recipe you've tried, each question answered, and each insight gained propel you forward on your path to a healthier, happier you. As you savour the flavours of your zero point meals, remember that every bite is a celebration of your commitment to well-being.

Here's to your continued journey into the world of Zero Point Cooking, where health and flavour coexist harmoniously. Your culinary adventure has just begun, and I wish you many more delicious discoveries ahead.

With gratitude,
  Lisa R. Ashley

FOOD JOURNAL

Breakfast	Servings	Calories
	Subtotal	

Snack		
	Subtotal	

Lunch		
	Subtotal	

Snack		
	Subtotal	

Dinner		
	Subtotal	

Snack		
	Subtotal	

Total Calories From Food

FITNESS ACTIVITY JOURNAL

	Duration	Calories

Total Calories From Fitness

NOTES

FOOD JOURNAL

Breakfast	Servings	Calories
		Subtotal

Snack		
		Subtotal

Lunch		
		Subtotal

Snack		
		Subtotal

Dinner		
		Subtotal

Snack		
		Subtotal

Total Calories From Food [   ]

FITNESS ACTIVITY JOURNAL

	Duration	Calories

Total Calories From Fitness [   ]

NOTES

FOOD JOURNAL

Breakfast	Servings	Calories
	Subtotal	

Snack		
	Subtotal	

Lunch		
	Subtotal	

Snack		
	Subtotal	

Dinner		
	Subtotal	

Snack		
	Subtotal	

Total Calories From Food [   ]

FITNESS ACTIVITY JOURNAL

	Duration	Calories

Total Calories From Fitness [   ]

NOTES

FOOD JOURNAL

Breakfast	Servings	Calories
	Subtotal	

Snack		
	Subtotal	

Lunch		
	Subtotal	

Snack		
	Subtotal	

Dinner		
	Subtotal	

Snack		
	Subtotal	

Total Calories From Food

FITNESS ACTIVITY JOURNAL

	Duration	Calories

Total Calories From Fitness

NOTES

Monday	Breakfast	Lunch	Dinner

Tuesday	Breakfast	Lunch	Dinner

Wednesday	Breakfast	Lunch	Dinner

Thursday	Breakfast	Lunch	Dinner

Friday	Breakfast	Lunch	Dinner

Saturday	Breakfast	Lunch	Dinner

Sunday	Breakfast	Lunch	Dinner

	Breakfast	Lunch	Dinner
Monday			

	Breakfast	Lunch	Dinner
Tuesday			

	Breakfast	Lunch	Dinner
Wednesday			

	Breakfast	Lunch	Dinner
Thursday			

	Breakfast	Lunch	Dinner
Friday			

	Breakfast	Lunch	Dinner
Saturday			

	Breakfast	Lunch	Dinner
Sunday			

Monday	Breakfast	Lunch	Dinner

Tuesday	Breakfast	Lunch	Dinner

Wednesday	Breakfast	Lunch	Dinner

Thursday	Breakfast	Lunch	Dinner

Friday	Breakfast	Lunch	Dinner

Saturday	Breakfast	Lunch	Dinner

Sunday	Breakfast	Lunch	Dinner

WRAP
CHICKEN
EGG SAL.
LOX

NOODLES
VEGGIE NOODLES

TOM SAUCE
SOUP
SPAGHETTI
EGGPLANT
ZITI W TURKEY

EGGS
SALAD
FRIED
SOFT BOILED
BOILED

Baabecued
Chicken
cooked
stir-fry
chik-sal.

TURKEY
GROUND
CHILIE
BURGERS
MEAT BALLS
ROASTED

CHEESE
STRING
SHRED
FETA
PARM.

cooked veggie
tomatos fryup
eggplant roasted
potato
potato beets

Beans
BAKED W CHEESE

beans + franks
bean soup

SOUP
BEAN
CHICKEN
BEEF
TOMATO
CORN
MUSHROOM
NOODLE
PEA
RATATOUILLE

pudding
boiled apple
hp2 jog.